Contents

Page

Foreword v

1 **Understanding the problem** 1
  What is diarrhoea? 1
  Acute and chronic diarrhoea 1
  Why is diarrhoea dangerous? 1
  How does diarrhoea cause dehydration? 2
  Treating a child who has diarrhoea 2
  ESSENTIAL SKILLS AND KNOWLEDGE: SECTION 1 4

2 **Home treatment of a child who has diarrhoea** 5
  Educating family members about home treatment of a child who has diarrhoea 5
  Three rules for home treatment of a child who has diarrhoea 6
  ESSENTIAL SKILLS AND KNOWLEDGE: SECTION 2 8

3 **Assessment by a health worker of a child who has diarrhoea** .. 9
  Examining the child 9
  Deciding on appropriate treatment 12
  ESSENTIAL SKILLS AND KNOWLEDGE: SECTION 3 13
  Examples of assessment 14

4 **Treatment by a health worker of a child who has diarrhoea** .. 18
  Ingredients of oral rehydration salts (ORS) 18
  How to prepare ORS solution 19
  How to treat a child who has diarrhoea 20
  Recording data on the child 24
  ESSENTIAL SKILLS AND KNOWLEDGE: SECTION 4 24

5 **Prevention of diarrhoea** 25
  Breast-feeding 25
  Improved weaning practices 26
  Use of plenty of clean water 27
  Hand-washing 27
  Use of latrines 28
  Proper disposal of the stools of young children 28
  Immunization against measles 29
  What health workers can do to support preventive practices 29
  ESSENTIAL SKILLS AND KNOWLEDGE: SECTION 5 30

6 **Things to remember about the treatment and prevention of diarrhoea** 31

Annexes

1 Diarrhoea Treatment Chart 32
2 How to treat diarrhoea at home (Mother's card) 37

Annexes (*continued*)

3 How to tell if a child is undernourished 38
4 What a health worker should do when packets of oral rehydration salts are not available 39
5 Oral rehydration using a nasogastric tube 42
6 Intravenous therapy for severe dehydration 43
7 Antibiotics used to treat diarrhoea caused by specific illnesses 47
8 Check-list of points of essential skills and knowledge 49

The treatment and prevention of acute diarrhoea

Practical guidelines

First edition 1985
Reprinted 1985, 1986
Second edition 1989

This book is also available in French and Spanish from WHO or from the sales agents listed on the inside back cover. Any part of the book may be copied or translated into other languages for non-profit-making purposes without prior permission from the World Health Organization, provided that two voucher copies of such translations are sent to the Organization. The Organization accepts no responsibility for the accuracy of any such translations. If a translation of the entire work is envisaged, inquiry should be made to the Office of Publications, World Health Organization, 1211 Geneva 27, Switzerland, to ensure that such a translation is not already available.

WHO welcomes comments on this guide and information on experience in its use; these should be addressed to:

Diarrhoeal Diseases Control Programme,
World Health Organization,
1211 Geneva 27,
Switzerland.

ISBN 92 4 154243 8
© World Health Organization 1989

PRINTED IN BELGIUM

6095/6602/6975

88/7719-Ceuterick-16 000

Foreword

This book is intended for health workers who are concerned with the prevention and treatment of diarrhoea, and for their supervisors and trainers. It is a revised and updated version of *Treatment and prevention of acute diarrhoea. Guidelines for the trainers of health workers* (Geneva, World Health Organization, 1985) and contains more information on prevention than the first edition. The guidelines form the technical basis of the module entitled *Treatment of diarrhoea* in the *Supervisory skills training course* of the WHO Diarrhoeal Diseases Control Programme.[1]

The book is divided into six sections. Each of the first five sections is followed by a list of points of essential skills and knowledge required by health workers for the prevention and treatment of acute diarrhoea. All 15 points of essential skills and knowledge are summarized in Annex 8. The Diarrhoea Treatment Chart, in Annex 1, summarizes the approach to management of diarrhoea explained in this book. The chart [1] may be adapted to local conditions and should be available to health workers for reference at all times.

[1] Available from: Diarrhoeal Diseases Control Programme, World Health Organization, 1211 Geneva 27, Switzerland.

1. Understanding the problem

What is diarrhoea?

The number of stools normally passed in a day varies with the diet and age of a person. In diarrhoea, stools contain more water than normal — they are often called loose or watery stools. They may also contain blood, in which case the diarrhoea is called dysentery.

Mothers usually know when their children have diarrhoea. When diarrhoea occurs mothers may say that the stools have a strong smell or pass noisily, as well as being loose and watery. By talking to mothers you can often find one or more useful local definitions of diarrhoea. In many societies, diarrhoea is defined as three or more loose or watery stools passed in a day.

Diarrhoea is most common in children, especially those between 6 months and 2 years of age. It is also common in babies under the age of 6 months who are drinking cow's milk or infant feeding formulas.

Frequent passing of normal stools is not diarrhoea.

Babies who are breast-fed often have stools that are soft; this is not diarrhoea.

Acute and chronic diarrhoea

Acute diarrhoea starts suddenly, and may continue for several days. It is caused by infection of the bowel. This book deals with the treatment and prevention of acute diarrhoea.

Chronic diarrhoea is diarrhoea that lasts for more than 2 weeks.

Why is diarrhoea dangerous?

Diarrhoea can cause undernutrition and death.

Death from acute diarrhoea or dysentery is most often caused by loss of a large amount of water and salt from the body. This loss is called dehydration.

Diarrhoea is more serious in people who are undernourished. It can cause undernutrition and can make existing undernutrition worse because during diarrhoea:

- nutrients are lost from the body;
- the person may not be hungry; and
- a mother may not feed a child who has diarrhoea. Some mothers may withhold food for some days after the diarrhoea is better.

To reduce this undernutrition, foods should be given to children who have diarrhoea as soon as they will eat.

How does diarrhoea cause dehydration?

The body normally takes in the water and salts it needs through drinks and food (input). It normally loses water and salts through stools, urine and sweat (output).

When the bowel is healthy, water and salts pass from the bowel into the blood. The water and salts can then be used by the body. When there is diarrhoea, the bowel does not work normally. Less water and salts pass into the blood, and more pass from the blood into the bowel. Thus, more than the normal amount of water and salts is passed out of the body, in the stools.

This larger than normal loss of water and salts from the body results in dehydration. It occurs when the output of water and salts is greater than the input. The more diarrhoea stools a person passes, the more water and salts he or she loses. Dehydration can be made worse by vomiting, which often accompanies diarrhoea.

Dehydration occurs faster in infants and young children, in hot climates, and when a person has fever.

Treating a child who has diarrhoea

The most important factors in the treatment of diarrhoea are:
- to prevent dehydration from occurring if possible;
- to treat dehydration quickly and well if it does occur; and
- to feed the child.

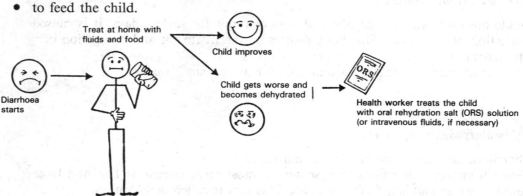

Treat at home with fluids and food

Child improves

Diarrhoea starts

Child gets worse and becomes dehydrated

Health worker treats the child with oral rehydration salt (ORS) solution (or intravenous fluids, if necessary)

Prevention of dehydration

Dehydration can usually be prevented in the home if the child drinks more fluids than usual as soon as the diarrhoea starts. A child should be given one of the fluids recommended for home treatment of diarrhoea in your area. Food-based fluids, for example, gruel, soup, or rice water, can be used. The fluids or solutions recommended in your area for preventing dehydration in the home will depend on:

- local traditions for the treatment of diarrhoea;
- the availability of a suitable food-based fluid;
- the availability of salt and sugar;
- the access of local people to health services; and
- the availability of oral rehydration salts (ORS).

Treatment of dehydration

If dehydration occurs, the child should be taken to a community health worker or health centre for treatment. The best treatment for dehydration is oral therapy with a solution made with oral rehydration salts (ORS). This treatment will be described in this book. This book talks about treating children, but the same treatment is also good for adults with diarrhoea. For treating dehydration, ORS should always be used if possible.

Feeding

While the child is ill with diarrhoea, he or she should frequently be offered small amounts of nutritious, easily digestible food. Feeding during the diarrhoea episode provides nutrients the child needs to be strong and to grow, and helps prevent weight loss. The extra fluids given to the child do not replace the need for food. After the diarrhoea has stopped, an extra meal each day for a week will help the child regain the weight lost during the illness.

Other treatments

There are no drugs available at present that will safely and effectively stop diarrhoea.

Antibiotics are not effective against most organisms that cause diarrhoea. They rarely help and can make some people sicker in the long term. Their indiscriminate use may increase the resistance of some disease-causing organisms to antibiotics. In addition, antibiotics are costly, so money is wasted. Therefore, antibiotics should not be used routinely. Their appropriate use for dysentery and cholera is described in Annex 7.

Adsorbants (such as kaolin, pectin, and activated charcoal) are not useful for the treatment of acute diarrhoea.

Antimotility drugs (such as tincture of opium) may be harmful, especially for children below 5 years of age. They temporarily reduce cramps and pain but delay the elimination from the body of the organisms that cause the diarrhoea, and may prolong the illness. They can be dangerous, and even fatal, if used incorrectly in infants.

ESSENTIAL SKILLS AND KNOWLEDGE: SECTION 1

The health worker should be able to do the following:

- Define diarrhoea in a way that is appropriate to his or her work setting.
- Distinguish between acute and chronic diarrhoea.
- Explain why diarrhoea is dangerous.
- Explain how diarrhoea causes dehydration.
- Describe the most important parts of the treatment of diarrhoea.

---

2. Home treatment of a child who has diarrhoea

Educating family members about home treatment of a child who has diarrhoea

Mothers and other family members can often treat children who have diarrhoea with fluids and foods that they have at home. Health workers can help by showing mothers how to do this.

There are three rules for treating diarrhoea in the home. Whenever a child gets diarrhoea, the mother (or any other family members who care for the child) should follow these rules. Briefly, the rules are:

- increase fluids;
- continue to feed the child;
- take the child to a health worker if he or she is not getting better.

These rules are also given in Treatment Plan A on page 21, and in *How to treat diarrhoea at home*, the mother's card given in Annex 2, page 37.

Steps for teaching families

Health workers should give information about home treatment to mothers and other family members whenever they have the opportunity, for example, when a mother comes for prenatal care or brings her child for immunization.

- Bear in mind the community's beliefs about diarrhoea and ways of treating it. Relate your advice to local practices, and use words that the mother will understand.
- Explain the three rules for treating diarrhoea at home.
- Show the mother what to do (for example, show her how much fluid to give the child after each stool).
- Use teaching aids that are familiar (for example, show the mother how to look for sunken eyes on her own child; use easily available containers to demonstrate how to mix ORS).
- Let the mother show you what she is learning (for example, how to feed the fluid with a spoon). In this way you will be sure that she can do it, and it will help her to remember.

- Ask the mother to tell you, in her own words, the things that she has learned but not practised. Again, this will help her to remember. For example, she can tell you what food she will give her child and how often.
- Ask the mother if she has any questions, and try to answer them.
- Ask her about any problems she may have in following the three rules. Listen to what she says and try to help her find a solution to any problem.
- Tell the mother what to expect (for example, how long it will take for her child to recover).

Three rules for home treatment of a child who has diarrhoea

RULE 1: GIVE THE CHILD MORE FLUIDS THAN USUAL

What fluids?

Give the recommended home fluid or food-based fluids, such as gruel, soup, or rice water.

If an infant is breast-fed — continue to breast-feed and try to do so more often than normal (at least every 3 hours).

If an infant is not breast-fed — dilute milk feed with twice the usual amount of water. Offer the milk feed at least every 3 hours.

How much fluid?

Give children under 2 years old approximately 50–100 ml ($\frac{1}{4}$–$\frac{1}{2}$ a large cup) of fluid after each loose stool. Give older children $\frac{1}{2}$ to 1 large cup. Adults should drink as much as they want.

RULE 2: CONTINUE TO FEED THE CHILD

What foods?

Weaning starts when a child is 4–6 months old.

Give a child of above this age foods with the highest amount of nutrients and calories relative to bulk. These foods should be mixes of cereal and locally available beans, or mixes of cereal and meat or fish. Add oil to these foods to make them richer in energy. Dairy products and eggs are also suitable. Fresh fruit juices and bananas are helpful because they help replace the potassium lost during diarrhoea.

In areas where vitamin A deficiency is common, foods that are rich in vitamin A are recommended for any child above 4–6 months old. These foods include liver, dairy products, and small, dried, whole fish. Red palm oil, which contains a very high amount of provitamin A, can also be added to foods.

6

Yellow vegetables (such as pumpkin, carrots and yellow sweet potatoes), dark green leafy vegetables (such as amaranth, spinach, and cassava leaves), and yellow fruits (such as mango and paw paw) also contain a lot of vitamin A. However, because many of these fruits and vegetables are bulky, it is preferable to give them in small amounts during and immediately after diarrhoea, and to give them only if the other foods that contain vitamin A are not available.

Avoid:

- High-fibre or bulky foods, such as coarse fruits and vegetables, fruit and vegetable peels, and whole grain cereals. These are hard to digest.
- Very dilute soups. These are recommended as fluids, but are not sufficient as foods because they fill up the child without providing sufficient nutrients.
- Foods with a lot of sugar. These foods can make diarrhoea worse.

How much food?

Encourage the child to eat as much as he or she wants. Offer food every 3 or 4 hours (five to seven times each day) or more often to a young child. Small, frequent feeds are best because they are more easily digested, and preferred by the child.

After the diarrhoea has stopped, give the child one extra meal each day for a week. This extra food helps the child regain the weight lost during the illness. Some children will continue to need extra foods to reach their pre-illness weight, or to reach a normal weight for their height.

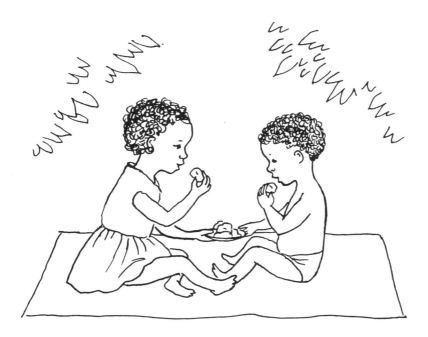

How to prepare the food

Prepare foods by cooking well, fermenting, mashing or grinding. This will make them easier to digest.

Give freshly prepared foods to minimize the chance of contamination. If previously prepared foods must be offered, first reheat them to boiling-point.

Why feed the child?

Starving a child who has diarrhoea can cause undernutrition, or make existing undernutrition worse. Mothers may withhold food, believing this will decrease the diarrhoea. But it is more important to give the child the nutrients he or she needs to stay strong and to grow. A strong child will resist illness better.

During and after diarrhoea give special attention to feeding the child nutritious food frequently. Even though absorption of nutrients from food is lessened somewhat during diarrhoea, most of the nutrients will be absorbed. Fluids given to the child do not replace the need for food.

RULE 3: TAKE YOUR CHILD TO THE HEALTH WORKER IF HE OR SHE IS NOT GETTING BETTER

If a child passes many stools, is very thirsty, or has sunken eyes, the child is probably dehydrated. The child may need more treatment than the mother can give at home.

The mother should take the child to a health worker if the child shows any of the following signs:

- passes many stools
- is very thirsty · These three signs suggest the child is dehydrated.
- has sunken eyes
- has a fever
- does not eat or drink normally
- seems not to be getting better.

ESSENTIAL SKILLS AND KNOWLEDGE: SECTION 2

- The health worker should be able to explain to family members the three rules for home treatment of diarrhoea. These are: to increase fluids; to continue to feed the child; and to take a child who is not getting better to the health worker.

---

3. Assessment by a health worker of a child who has diarrhoea

Examining the child

When a child comes to a health worker or health centre because of diarrhoea, the first step is to assess the child for signs of dehydration. The health worker should also ask if there is diarrhoea when a child comes with an illness, such as measles, that is often accompanied by diarrhoea.

A list of the questions that the health worker should ask, the conditions to feel for, and the things to look for are presented here and given on the assessment chart shown on page 10, and in Annex 1.

As you read this section, refer to the assessment chart on page 10. When you examine a child, note your findings and see into which column on the assessment chart they fall.

Ask the following questions

- How many liquid stools per day has the child been passing?
  For how long has the child had diarrhoea?
  Is there blood (more than 1 or 2 streaks) in the stools?

- Has the child been vomiting?
  If so, has the child vomited more than a small amount?
  How frequently has the child vomited?

- Is the child able to drink?
  If so, is the child thirstier than usual?

- Has the child passed urine in the last 6 hours?
  If so, is it a normal amount or a small amount?
  Is it darker than usual?

HOW TO ASSESS YOUR PATIENT

	FOR DEHYDRATION			FOR OTHER PROBLEMS
	A	**B**	**C**	
1. ASK ABOUT: DIARRHOEA	Less than 4 liquid stools per day	4 to 10 liquid stools per day	More than 10 liquid stools per day	Longer than 14 days duration / Blood in the stool
VOMITING	None or a small amount	Some	Very frequent	
THIRST	Normal	Greater than normal	Unable to drink	
URINE	Normal	A small amount, dark	No urine for 6 hours	
2. LOOK AT: CONDITION	Well, alert	Unwell, sleepy or irritable	Very sleepy, unconscious, floppy or having fits	Severe undernutrition
TEARS	Present	Absent	Absent	
EYES	Normal	Sunken	Very dry and sunken	
MOUTH and TONGUE	Wet	Dry	Very dry	
BREATHING	Normal	Faster than normal	Very fast and deep	
3. FEEL: SKIN	A pinch goes back quickly	A pinch goes back slowly	A pinch goes back very slowly	
PULSE	Normal	Faster than normal	Very fast, weak, or you cannot feel it	
FONTANELLE (in infants)	Normal	Sunken	Very sunken	
4. TAKE TEMPERATURE				Fever – 38.5°C (or 101°F) or greater
5. WEIGH IF POSSIBLE	Loss of less than 25 grams for each kilogram of weight	Loss of 25-100 grams for each kilogram of weight	Loss of more than 100 grams for each kilogram of weight	
6. DECIDE	The patient has **no signs of dehydration**	If the patient has 2 or more of these signs, he has **some dehydration**	If the patient has 2 or more of these danger signs, he has **severe dehydration**	
	Use Plan A	**Use Plan B**	**Use Plan C**	

IF YOUR PATIENT HAS:	THEN:
Blood in the stool and diarrhoea for less than 14 days	Treat with an appropriate oral antibiotic for shigella dysentery. If this child is also – dehydrated, – severely undernourished, or – less than 1 year of age, reassess the child's progress in 24 - 48 hours. For the severely undernourished child, also refer for treatment of severe undernutrition.
Diarrhoea for longer than 14 days with or without blood	Continue feeding and refer for treatment.
Severe undernutrition	
Fever – 38.5°C (or 101°F) or greater	Show the mother how to cool the child with a wet cloth and fanning. Look for and treat other causes (for example, pneumonia, malaria).

10

Look for the following conditions

- What is the child's general condition?
- Is the child
    - well and alert?
    - unwell, sleepy, or irritable?
    - very sleepy, floppy, or unconscious?
    - having fits?
    - severely undernourished? (See Annex 3, *How to tell if a child is undernourished*, on page 38).
- Does the child have tears when he or she cries?
- Are the child's eyes normal, sunken, or very dry and sunken?
- Are the child's mouth and tongue wet, dry, or very dry?
- Is the child's breathing normal, faster than normal, or very fast and deep?

Feel for the following

- When the skin is pinched, does it go back quickly, slowly, or very slowly (taking longer than 2 seconds)? In a baby, the health worker should pinch the skin of the abdomen or thigh.
    Note: Pinching the skin may give misleading information if a child is either undernourished or obese.
    - In a severely undernourished child, the skin may go back slowly, even if the child is not dehydrated.
    - In an obese child, the skin may go back quickly even if he or she is dehydrated.
- Can the pulse be felt?
    If so, is it normal, faster than normal, very fast, or weak?
- Is the fontanelle (the soft spot on top of the head of infants) normal, sunken, or very sunken?
    Note: This is a helpful sign only in children whose fontanelle is not yet closed (usually children under 12 months old).

Weigh the child, if a weighing scale is available

- If a scale is available, carefully weigh the child unclothed or lightly clothed.
    If the child has been weighed routinely and the weight recorded, compare the child's present weight with the last recorded weight.
    Has there been any loss of weight during the diarrhoea?
    If so, were less than 25 g lost for each kg of the child's weight?
    Were 25–100 g lost for each kg of the child's weight?
    Were more than 100 g lost for each kg of weight?

Note: Loss of fluid causes loss of weight. Assessing weight loss is useful if a health worker has a very accurate scale and knows how to use the scale correctly. If a child has been weighed recently, the weight loss will give some idea of how much fluid has been lost. Weighing the child again later can help to assess progress. However, it is more useful to rely on clinical signs than on measuring weight loss to make a judgement about dehydration.

- If a scale is not available, rely on observing clinical signs, and do not delay treatment.

Take the child's temperature

- Does the child have a fever (a temperature of more than 38.5 °C)?
  Note: Rectal temperature should be taken, if the health worker is used to that procedure and is able to disinfect the thermometer after each use. Otherwise, the axillary (armpit) temperature should be taken.

Deciding on appropriate treatment

After the examination, decide how to treat the child.

- Recall your findings while you were examining the child and look at the chart on page 10.
- If the child has any of the signs in the column labelled "FOR OTHER PROBLEMS", specific treatment is needed in addition to any treatment given for dehydration. Details of the specific treatment are given at the foot of the "FOR OTHER PROBLEMS" column.
- Determine the degree of dehydration:
  — Look at Column C. If two or more of the signs listed in Column C are present, conclude that the child has severe dehydration.
  — If two or more signs from Column C are not present, look at Column B. If two or more of the signs listed in Column B are present, conclude that the child has some dehydration.
  — If two or more signs from Column B are not present, conclude that the child has no signs of dehydration.
- Select the appropriate treatment plan:
  — For no signs of dehydration, select Treatment Plan A — *To treat diarrhoea* (see page 21).
  — For some dehydration, select Treatment Plan B — *To treat dehydration* (see page 22).
  — For severe dehydration, select Treatment Plan C — *To treat severe dehydration quickly* (see page 23).

These treatment plans are also given in Annex 1.

12

Two examples of how health workers have selected the appropriate treatment plans for children with diarrhoea are given on pages 14 and 16.

ESSENTIAL SKILLS AND KNOWLEDGE : SECTION 3

The health worker should be able to do the following:
- Ask, look, and feel for signs of dehydration, and check for problems other than dehydration.
- Select the appropriate treatment plan using the assessment chart given on page 10 and in Annex 1.

Examples of assessment

Example 1

A mother took her 5-month-old son, Sione, to a health worker because he had diarrhoea. The health worker asked, looked, and felt for signs of dehydration. On page 15 is the "*How to assess your patient*" chart with the health worker's findings circled.

Since Sione had no signs from Column C and more than two signs from Column B, the health worker concluded that Sione had some dehydration. The health worker selected Treatment Plan B to treat the dehydration.

HOW TO ASSESS YOUR PATIENT

FOR DEHYDRATION

	A	B	C	FOR OTHER PROBLEMS
1. ASK ABOUT: DIARRHOEA	Less than 4 liquid stools per day	4 to 10 liquid stools per day	More than 10 liquid stools per day	Longer than 14 days duration / Blood in the stool
VOMITING	None or a small amount	Some	Very frequent	
THIRST	Normal	Greater than normal	Unable to drink	
URINE	Normal	A small amount, dark	No urine for 6 hours	
2. LOOK AT: CONDITION	Well, alert	Unwell, sleepy or irritable	Very sleepy, unconscious, floppy or having fits	Severe undernutrition
TEARS	Present	Absent	Absent	
EYES	Normal	Sunken	Very dry and sunken	
MOUTH and TONGUE	Wet	Dry	Very dry	
BREATHING	Normal	Faster than normal	Very fast and deep	
3. FEEL: SKIN	A pinch goes back quickly	A pinch goes back slowly	A pinch goes back very slowly	
PULSE	Normal	Faster than normal	Very fast, weak, or you cannot feel it	
FONTANELLE (in infants)	Normal	Sunken	Very sunken	
4. TAKE TEMPERATURE				Fever – 38.5°C (or 101°F) or greater
5. WEIGH IF POSSIBLE	Loss of less than 25 grams for each kilogram of weight	Loss of 25-100 grams for each kilogram of weight	Loss of more than 100 grams for each kilogram of weight	
6. DECIDE	The patient has no signs of dehydration	If the patient has 2 or more of these signs, he has **some dehydration**	If the patient has 2 or more of these danger signs, he has **severe dehydration**	
	Use Plan A	**Use Plan B**	**Use Plan C**	

FOR OTHER PROBLEMS

IF YOUR PATIENT HAS:	THEN:
Blood in the stool and diarrhoea for less than 14 days	Treat with an appropriate oral antibiotic for shigella dysentery. If this child is also – dehydrated, – severely undernourished, or – less than 1 year of age, reassess the child's progress in 24 - 48 hours. For the severely undernourished child, also refer for treatment of severe undernutrition.
Diarrhoea for longer than 14 days with or without blood	Continue feeding and refer for treatment.
Severe undernutrition	
Fever – 38.5°C (or 101°F) or greater	Show the mother how to cool the child with a wet cloth and fanning. Look for and treat other causes (for example, pneumonia, malaria).

Example 2

A mother took her 3-year-old daughter, Rania, to a clinic because she had diarrhoea. The clinic worker asked, looked and felt for signs of dehydration. On page 17 is the "*How to assess your patient*" chart with the health worker's findings circled.

Because Rania had blood in her stools and had had diarrhoea for less than 14 days, the clinic worker suspected dysentery and gave the mother an appropriate antibiotic for the child. (This was trimethoprim + sulfamethoxazole, to which most shigellae in the area were known to be sensitive.) Because Rania had a fever, the clinic worker showed the mother how to cool her with a wet cloth and fanning. The clinic worker did not find any apparent cause for the fever.

Since Rania had no signs from Column C and only one sign from Column B, the clinic worker decided that she had no signs of dehydration. The clinic worker selected Treatment Plan A, to treat diarrhoea at home, and to prevent Rania from becoming dehydrated.

HOW TO ASSESS YOUR PATIENT

FOR DEHYDRATION

	A	B	C
1. ASK ABOUT: DIARRHOEA	Less than 4 liquid stools per day	4 to 10 liquid stools per day	More than 10 liquid stools per day
VOMITING	None or a small amount	Some	Very frequent
THIRST	Normal	Greater than normal	Unable to drink
URINE	Normal	A small amount, dark	No urine for 6 hours
2. LOOK AT: CONDITION	Well, alert	Unwell, sleepy or irritable	Very sleepy, unconscious, floppy or having fits
TEARS	Present	Absent	Absent
EYES	Normal	Sunken	Very dry and sunken
MOUTH and TONGUE	Wet	Dry	Very dry
BREATHING	Normal	Faster than normal	Very fast and deep
3. FEEL: SKIN	A pinch goes back quickly	A pinch goes back slowly	A pinch goes back very slowly
PULSE	Normal	Faster than normal	Very fast, weak, or you cannot feel it
FONTANELLE (in infants)	Normal	Sunken	Very sunken
4. TAKE TEMPERATURE			
5. WEIGH IF POSSIBLE	Loss of less than 25 grams for each kilogram of weight	Loss of 25-100 grams for each kilogram of weight	Loss of more than 100 grams for each kilogram of weight
6. DECIDE	The patient has **no** signs of dehydration	If the patient has 2 or more of these signs, he has **some** dehydration	If the patient has 2 or more of these danger signs, he has **severe** dehydration
	Use Plan A	Use Plan B	Use Plan C

FOR OTHER PROBLEMS

Longer than 14 days duration
Blood in the stool

Severe undernutrition

Fever – 38.5°C (or 101°F) or greater

IF YOUR PATIENT HAS:	THEN:
Blood in the stool and diarrhoea for less than 14 days	Treat with an appropriate oral antibiotic for shigella dysentery. If this child is also – dehydrated, – severely undernourished, or – less than 1 year of age, reassess the child's progress in 24 - 48 hours. For the severely undernourished child, also refer for treatment of severe undernutrition.
Diarrhoea for longer than 14 days with or without blood	Continue feeding and refer for treatment.
Severe undernutrition	
Fever – 38.5°C (or 101°F) or greater	Show the mother how to cool the child with a wet cloth and fanning. Look for and treat other causes (for example, pneumonia, malaria).

17

4. Treatment by a health worker of a child who has diarrhoea

Dehydration is treated with ORS solution. All health workers should have the skill to prepare ORS solution from water and oral rehydration salts (ORS).

Ingredients of oral rehydration salts (ORS)

Oral rehydration salts often come in packets containing the following ingredients:

Ingredient	Amount
Sodium chloride (common salt)	3.5 g
Glucose (a form of sugar)	20 g
Trisodium citrate, dihydrate	2.9 g
or sodium bicarbonate (baking soda)	2.5 g
Potassium chloride	1.5 g

Packets containing these ingredients in these amounts are made for mixing with one litre of drinking-water.

Note: Some packets of ORS are made for smaller volumes of water; they contain smaller amounts of the same ingredients. It is critical that the correct amount of water is used to mix with any packet. If not enough water is used, the solution will be too strong, and may be dangerous. If too much water is used, the solution will be too dilute and may not be as effective.

When ORS packets are not available, oral rehydration solution can be made by following the instructions in Annex 4 (page 39).

How to prepare ORS solution

Wash your hands with soap and water.

Pour all the powder from one packet of ORS into a clean container. Use whatever container is available such as a jar, bowl or bottle.

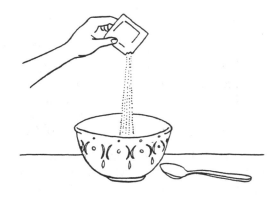

Measure 1 litre of clean water (or the correct amount for the packet used). It is best to boil and cool the water before use, but if this is not possible, use the cleanest drinking-water available.

Pour the water into the container. Mix well with a clean spoon until the powder is completely dissolved.

Taste the solution so you know what it tastes like.

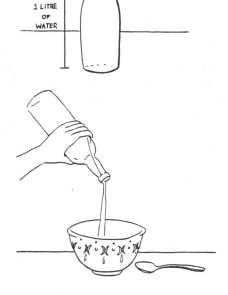

Mix fresh ORS solution each day in a clean container. Keep the container covered. The solution can be kept and used for one day (24 hours). Throw away any solution remaining from the day before.

How to treat a child who has diarrhoea

On the basis of the assessment of the degree of dehydration of the child, the health worker should have selected one of the following treatment plans:

Treatment Plan A — *To treat diarrhoea*
Treatment Plan B — *To treat dehydration*
Treatment Plan C — *To treat severe dehydration quickly*
(For Treatment Plan C see also Annexes 5 and 6 on pages 42 and 43).

Some health workers may not have the skills or the necessary supplies to perform all the steps listed in each treatment plan. A supervisor or trainer must determine which procedures can be performed by a health worker in a community setting, and which can only be performed by a health worker in a health facility. Then the supervisor or trainer must give each type of health worker the training and supplies needed to carry out the treatment correctly.

The health worker will then follow the treatment plan selected. He or she may also need to treat any other problems that have been identified. In all cases, the health worker should first compliment the mother on bringing her child for care.

Many mothers will expect to be given a medicine to stop the diarrhoea. But it is the dehydration that is the main cause of death. It is necessary to take time to explain to the mother that it is most important to treat dehydration by replacing the fluids lost, and to continue feeding the child. In cases of dysentery and cholera, treatment with antibiotics may be necessary (see Annex 7, page 47). In most cases, however, treatment with drugs will not help. In nearly all cases, diarrhoea will stop without treatment with drugs.

Before going home all mothers should be taught the three rules for home treatment of diarrhoea given on pages 6–8 and in Treatment Plan A. Even children who are treated at the facility according to Treatment Plan B or C will require treatment according to Plan A when their condition has improved.

Remember

All children with diarrhoea will be treated with Plan A, that is, both:
- children who have not developed signs of dehydration, and
- children who have already been treated for dehydration, and have improved.

Remember that it is important to give ORS solution in small amounts at a steady pace (a teaspoonful every 1–2 minutes), and that after receiving ORS solution for 4 to 6 hours (on Plan B), most children will improve sufficiently to be treated according to Plan A.

TREATMENT PLAN A
TO TREAT DIARRHOEA

EXPLAIN THE THREE RULES FOR TREATING DIARRHOEA AT HOME:

1. GIVE YOUR CHILD MORE FLUIDS THAN USUAL TO PREVENT DEHYDRATION.
   SUITABLE FLUIDS INCLUDE:
   - The recommended home fluid or food-based fluids, such as gruel, soup, or rice water.
   - Breast milk or milk feeds prepared with twice the usual amount of water.

2. GIVE YOUR CHILD FOOD:
   - Give freshly prepared foods. Recommended foods are mixes of cereal and beans, or cereal and meat or fish. Add a few drops of oil to the food, if possible.
   - Give fresh fruit juices or bananas to provide potassium.
   - Offer food every 3 or 4 hours (6 times a day) or more often for very young children.
   - Encourage the child to eat as much as he or she wants.
   - Cook and mash or grind food well so it will be easier to digest.
   - After the diarrhoea stops, give one extra meal each day for a week, or until the child has regained normal weight.

3. TAKE YOUR CHILD TO THE HEALTH WORKER IF THE CHILD HAS ANY OF THE FOLLOWING:
   - passes many stools ⎫
   - is very thirsty   ⎬ These 3 signs suggest your child is dehydrated.
   - has sunken eyes   ⎭
   - has a fever
   - does not eat or drink normally
   - seems not to be getting better.

TEACH THE MOTHER HOW TO USE ORS SOLUTION AT HOME, IF:
   - The mother cannot come back if the diarrhoea gets worse.
   - It is national policy to give ORS to all children who see a health worker for diarrhoea treatment, or
   - Her child has been on Plan B, to prevent dehydration from coming back.

SHOW HER HOW TO MIX AND GIVE ORS.

SHOW HER HOW MUCH TO GIVE:
   - 50-100 ml (¼ to ½ large cup) of ORS solution after each stool for a child under 2 years old.
   - 100-200 ml (½ to 1 large cup) for older children.
   - Adults should drink as much as they want.

TELL HER IF THE CHILD VOMITS, wait 10 minutes. Then continue giving the solution but more slowly — a spoonful every 2-3 minutes.

GIVE HER ENOUGH PACKETS FOR 2 DAYS.

Note: While a child is getting ORS, he or she should be given breast milk or dilute milk feeds and should be offered food. Food-based fluids or a salt and sugar solution should *NOT* be given in addition to ORS.

EXPLAIN HOW SHE CAN PREVENT DIARRHOEA BY:

Giving only breast milk for the first 4-6 months and continuing to breast-feed for at least the first year.

Introducing clean, nutritious weaning foods at 4-6 months.

Giving her child freshly prepared and well-cooked food and clean drinking-water.

Having all family members wash their hands with soap after defecating, and before eating or preparing food.

Having all family members use a latrine.

Quickly disposing of the stool of a young child by putting it into a latrine or by burying it.

TREATMENT PLAN B
TO TREAT DEHYDRATION

1. AMOUNT OF ORS SOLUTION TO GIVE IN FIRST 4 TO 6 HOURS

Patient's age	2 4 6 8 10 12 18 2 months →	3 4 6 8 15 ← years →	adult
Patient's weight in kilograms	3 5 7 9 11 13 15 20 30 40 50		
Give this much solution for 4-6 hours	in ml	200-400	400-600	600-800	800-1000	1000-2000	2000-4000
	in local unit of measure						

- Use the patient's age only when you do not know the weight.

NOTE: ENCOURAGE THE MOTHER TO CONTINUE BREAST-FEEDING.

If the patient wants more ORS, give more.

If the eyelids become puffy, stop ORS and give other fluids. If diarrhoea continues, use ORS again when the puffiness is gone.

If the child vomits, wait 10 minutes and then continue giving ORS, but more slowly.

2. IF THE MOTHER CAN REMAIN AT THE HEALTH CENTRE

- Show her how much solution to give her child.
- Show her how to give it — a spoonful every 1 to 2 minutes.
- Check from time to time to see if she has problems.

3. AFTER 4 TO 6 HOURS, REASSESS THE CHILD USING THE ASSESSMENT CHART. THEN CHOOSE THE SUITABLE TREATMENT PLAN.

Note: If a child will continue on Plan B, tell the mother to offer small amounts of food.

If the child is under 12 months, tell the mother to:
- continue breast-feeding or
- if she does not breast-feed, give 100-200 ml of clean water before continuing ORS.

4. IF THE MOTHER MUST LEAVE ANY TIME BEFORE COMPLETING TREATMENT PLAN B

- Give her enough ORS packets for 2 days and show her how to prepare the fluid.
- Show her how much ORS to give to finish the 4-6 hour treatment at home.
- Tell her to give the child as much ORS and other fluids as he or she wants after the 4-6 hour treatment is finished.
- Tell her to offer the child small amounts of food every 3-4 hours.
- Tell her to bring the child back to the health worker if the child has any of the following:
  - passes many stools
  - is very thirsty   These 3 signs suggest the child is dehydrated.
  - has sunken eyes
  - has a fever
  - does not eat or drink normally
  - seems not to be getting better.

22

TREATMENT PLAN C
TO TREAT SEVERE
DEHYDRATION QUICKLY

Follow the arrows. If the answer to the questions is 'yes', go across. If it is 'no', go down.

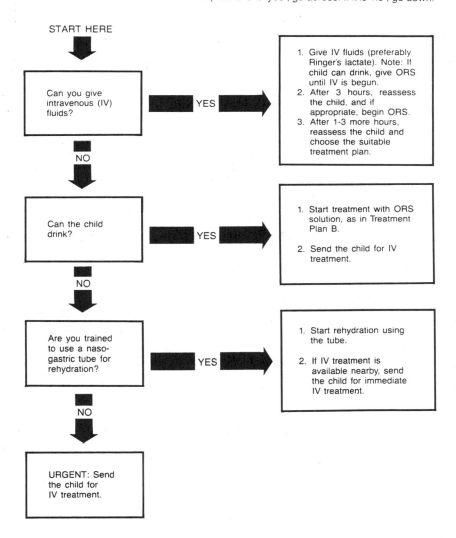

START HERE

Can you give intravenous (IV) fluids?

YES

1. Give IV fluids (preferably Ringer's lactate). Note: If child can drink, give ORS until IV is begun.
2. After 3 hours, reassess the child, and if appropriate, begin ORS.
3. After 1-3 more hours, reassess the child and choose the suitable treatment plan.

NO

Can the child drink?

YES

1. Start treatment with ORS solution, as in Treatment Plan B.
2. Send the child for IV treatment.

NO

Are you trained to use a naso-gastric tube for rehydration?

YES

1. Start rehydration using the tube.
2. If IV treatment is available nearby, send the child for immediate IV treatment.

NO

URGENT: Send the child for IV treatment.

NOTE: If the child is above 2 years of age and cholera is known to be currently occurring in your area, suspect cholera and give an appropriate oral antibiotic once the child is alert.

23

If a child begins to vomit while being given ORS solution, wait 10 minutes then continue giving the solution, but more slowly. Some children may want to drink too quickly. This may make them vomit.

Recording data on the child

Health workers in the community and in the health facility should keep a record on each child who comes for treatment or to use a service.

At a minimum, each child must be identified in the records by:

- name
- age (or date of birth)
- date of visit
- reason for visit
- diagnosis
- type of treatment or service provided.

From this information a health worker can count the number of episodes of diarrhoea treated in children of less than 5 years each month, and the number of children given other services.

Additional data that may be recorded include the sex of the child, the address (the health worker may want to ask the distance the child has travelled to receive treatment), information from the physical examination, and whether the child has watery diarrhoea or dysentery.

These records should be kept for periodic review by the supervisor in order to monitor the use of various services and to help plan future use.

The forms used for patient records may be different in different health facilities or areas. It is important that the form includes the minimum data and is easy to understand and fill in. If existing record-keeping systems in a health area do not include the minimum information, the supervisor might modify them to include that information, or create new forms. If the same form is used by all health workers in an area, it will be easier to collect data when monitoring the use of services.

ESSENTIAL SKILLS AND KNOWLEDGE: SECTION 4

The health worker should be able to do the following:

- Demonstrate how to prepare ORS solution correctly.
- Give oral rehydration therapy to dehydrated children.
- Give intravenous rehydration therapy to children with severe dehydration or refer then for this treatment.
- Teach mothers how to continue treatment at home.
- Keep appropriate records of treatment given.

---

5. Prevention of diarrhoea

An important job of the health worker is to help prevent diarrhoea by convincing and helping community members to adopt certain preventive practices and to continue to practise them. These preventive practices are:

- breast-feeding
- improved weaning practices
- use of plenty of clean water
- hand-washing
- use of latrines
- proper disposal of the stools of young children
- immunization against measles.

The health worker can teach, encourage, and set a good example to influence community members to adopt these preventive practices.

Some simple facts that people in the community should know about each preventive practice are presented on the following pages.

Breast-feeding

- Mothers should give only breast milk to their babies for the first 4–6 months and then some breast milk, along with the other foods, for up to at least one year.
- To breast-feed comfortably and safely, mothers should:
  - not give their babies extra fluids, such as water, sugar water, or milk formula, especially in the early days of life;
  - start breast-feeding as soon as possible after the baby is born;
  - breast-feed on demand (increased sucking increases milk supply);
  - express milk manually to avoid engorgement of the breasts during periods of separation from the baby.
- If the mother works outside the home and it is not possible for her to take the baby with her, she should breast-feed before leaving home, on returning at night and at any other time when she is with the baby.

- A mother should continue breast-feeding when her baby is ill, and after the illness. This is especially important if the baby has diarrhoea.

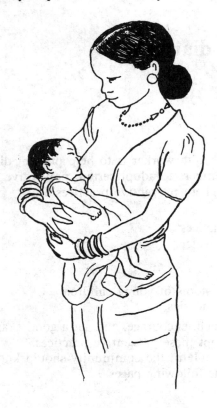

Improved weaning practices

- Clean, nutritious weaning foods should be introduced when a child is about 4–6 months old. Initially soft mashed foods are best.
- A child's diet should become increasingly varied and should include: the staple food of the community (usually a cereal or root); beans or peas; some food from animals, for example, milk products, eggs and meat; and green leafy vegetables or orange vegetables.
- A child should also be given some fruit or fruit juice, and some oil or fat should be added to the weaning food.
- Family members should wash their hands before preparing weaning food, and before feeding a baby.
- Food should be prepared in a clean place, using clean pots and utensils.
- Uncooked food should be washed in clean water before it is eaten.

- Cooked food should be eaten while it is still hot, or thoroughly re-heated before eating.
- Foods that are being kept should be covered and, if possible, refrigerated.

Use of plenty of clean water

- Water should be collected from the cleanest available source.
- Water sources should be protected by: keeping animals away; locating latrines more than 10 metres away from the source, and downhill; and digging drainage ditches uphill from the source to channel storm-water away.
- Water should be collected and stored in clean containers. It should be taken from the storage container with a clean, long-handled dipper.
- Water used for making food or drinks for young children should be boiled.

Hand-washing

- All family members should wash their hands well:
  — after cleaning a child who has defecated, and after disposing of a child's stool
  — after defecation
  — before preparing food
  — before eating
  — before feeding a child.
- An adult or older sibling should wash the hands of young children.

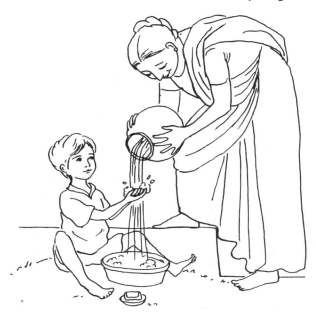

Use of latrines

- All families should have a clean and functioning latrine. The latrine should be used by all family members who are old enough to use it.
- The latrine should be kept clean by regular washing of dirty surfaces.
- If there is no latrine, family members should:
    - defecate at a distance from the house, paths, or areas where children play, and at least 10 metres from the water supply
    - avoid going barefoot to defecate
    - not allow a child to visit the defecation area alone.

Proper disposal of the stools of young children

- Quickly collect the stool of a young child or baby, wrap it in a leaf or newspaper, and bury it or put it into the latrine.
- Young children should be helped to defecate into an easily cleaned container. The stool should then be put into a latrine and the container washed out. Alternatively, the child can defecate onto a surface such as a newspaper or large leaf, and this can be put into a latrine.
- A child who has defecated should be cleaned promptly, and the child's hands should be washed.

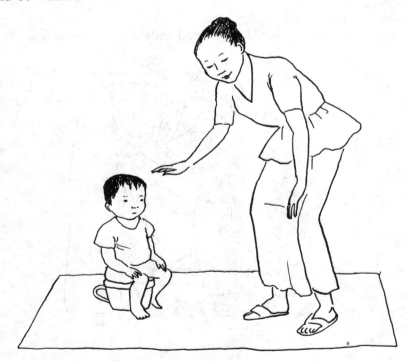

Immunization against measles

- Children should be immunized against measles as soon after 9 months of age as possible.

What health workers can do to support preventive practices

1. Use good educational techniques

Messages about ways to prevent diarrhoea should be brief and clearly relevant to the person or group with whom the health worker is talking. The health worker should only discuss a few messages at a time. If health workers use good educational techniques, they will be more effective in helping community members understand the benefits of the preventive practices. The steps for teaching families about home treatment of diarrhoea given on pages 5-6 are also useful when teaching about prevention.

2. Set a good example

Health workers should always 'practise what they preach' about prevention. What a person does always sends a more powerful message than what the person says.

3. Participate in community projects to improve preventive practices

In cooperation with existing community groups, health workers can use their knowledge of ways to prevent diarrhoea to help plan useful projects. Some examples of projects that could be carried out with limited community resources, and that would significantly benefit many community members, include:
- buying soap in bulk for the community
- improving water sources
- designating and supporting a builder to build family latrines
- gardening to produce better and cheaper ingredients for weaning food.

4. Support breast-feeding

A health worker who attends the birth of a baby can help the mother begin breast-feeding by doing the things listed below. Health workers can also encourage traditional birth attendants or family members attending a birth to do these things.
- Give the infant to the mother to begin breast-feeding immediately after delivery, or as soon as possible after delivery.

- Let the mother and infant stay in the same room, or bring the infant to breast-feed when hungry.
- Do not give feeds other than breast milk to a newborn baby.
- Show the mother the best way to breast-feed, and how to avoid problems with breast-feeding.

Health workers can encourage mothers who are breast-feeding to meet together to discuss any problems they may be having. This is a breast-feeding support group.

5. Build and maintain a latrine at the health facility

A clean, functioning latrine at the health facility will be an example to people coming for health services. It should be properly maintained and kept clean, so that community members see how a latrine should work.

6. Tell community members where the clean water sources are and how to improve water sources

Probably some of the sources of water in a community can be improved by taking simple measures such as those listed below. Community members may want to make improvements to water sources if health workers can tell them exactly what should be done, for example:
- Build a fence or wall around the water source to keep animals away.
- Dig drainage ditches uphill from an open well to prevent storm-water from flowing into it.
- Do not allow washing in the water source.
- Do not allow children to play in or around the water source.
- Do not locate latrines uphill from, or within 10 metres of, the water source.
- Install a simple pulley device and bucket to make it easier to raise water from a well.

ESSENTIAL SKILLS AND KNOWLEDGE: SECTION 5

The health worker should be able to do the following:
- Describe what families can do to prevent diarrhoea, including:
    - breast-feeding;
    - improved weaning practices;
    - the use of plenty of clean water;
    - hand-washing;
    - the use of latrines;
    - proper disposal of the stools of young children;
    - immunization against measles.
- List several things that health workers can do to support preventive practices.

---

6. Things to remember about the treatment and prevention of diarrhoea

- The most important problem to treat in a patient with diarrhoea is dehydration.
- Family members should be taught how to treat diarrhoea. The three rules for home treatment of a child with diarrhoea are:
  1. Give the child more fluids than usual.
  2. Continue to feed the child.
  3. Take a child who is not getting better to the health worker.
- When a child with diarrhoea comes to a health worker, the health worker should:
  - Ask, look and feel for signs of dehydration.
  - Check for problems other than dehydration (for example, dysentery).
  - Select a treatment plan.
  - Give oral rehydration therapy to children with dehydration.
  - Give intravenous rehydration therapy to children with severe dehydration, or refer them for this treatment.
  - Refer or give appropriate treatment for any other problem found.
- The health worker should use the Diarrhoea Treatment Chart given in Annex 1 when assessing and treating children with diarrhoea.
- The health worker should be able to describe what families can do to prevent diarrhoea, including breast-feeding, improved weaning practices, use of plenty of clean water, hand-washing, use of latrines, proper disposal of the stools of young children, and immunization against measles.
- Some things that health workers can do to support preventive practices include:
  - Using good educational techniques.
  - Setting a good example.
  - Participating in community projects to improve preventive practices.
  - Supporting breast-feeding.
  - Building and maintaining a latrine at the health facility.
  - Telling community members where the clean water sources are and how to improve water sources.

Annex 1. Diarrhoea Treatment Chart

Note: The Assessment Chart opposite and Treatment Plans A, B, and C (on pages 34-36) all appear on the WHO Diarrhoea Treatment Chart. This is a poster-sized chart for hanging on the wall. It is available from Diarrhoeal Diseases Control, World Health Organization, 1211 Geneva 27, Switzerland, and from WHO Regional Offices.

HOW TO ASSESS YOUR PATIENT

FOR DEHYDRATION | FOR OTHER PROBLEMS

		A	B	C	FOR OTHER PROBLEMS
1 ASK ABOUT:	DIARRHOEA	Less than 4 liquid stools per day	4 to 10 liquid stools per day	More than 10 liquid stools per day	Longer than 14 days duration / Blood in the stool
	VOMITING	None or a small amount	Some	Very frequent	
	THIRST	Normal	Greater than normal	Unable to drink	
	URINE	Normal	A small amount, dark	No urine for 6 hours	
2 LOOK AT:	CONDITION	Well, alert	Unwell, sleepy or irritable	Very sleepy, unconscious, floppy or having fits	Severe undernutrition
	TEARS	Present	Absent	Absent	
	EYES	Normal	Sunken	Very dry and sunken	
	MOUTH and TONGUE	Wet	Dry	Very dry	
	BREATHING	Normal	Faster than normal	Very fast and deep	
3 FEEL:	SKIN PULSE	A pinch goes back quickly / Normal	A pinch goes back slowly / Faster than normal	A pinch goes back very slowly / Very fast, weak, or you cannot feel it	
	FONTANELLE (in infants)	Normal	Sunken	Very sunken	
4 TAKE TEMPERATURE					Fever – 38.5°C (or 101°F) or greater
5 WEIGH IF POSSIBLE		Loss of less than 25 grams for each kilogram of weight	Loss of 25-100 grams for each kilogram of weight	Loss of more than 100 grams for each kilogram of weight	
6 DECIDE		The patient has **no** signs of dehydration	If the patient has 2 or more of these signs, he has **some** dehydration	If the patient has 2 or more of these danger signs, he has **severe dehydration**	
		Use Plan A	**Use Plan B**	**Use Plan C**	

IF YOUR PATIENT HAS:	THEN:
Blood in the stool and diarrhoea for less than 14 days	Treat with an appropriate oral antibiotic for shigella dysentery. If this child is also – dehydrated, – severely undernourished, or – less than 1 year of age, reassess the child's progress in 24 - 48 hours. For the severely undernourished child, also refer for treatment of severe undernutrition.
Diarrhoea for longer than 14 days with or without blood	Continue feeding and refer for treatment.
Severe undernutrition	
Fever – 38.5°C (or 101°F) or greater	Show the mother how to cool the child with a wet cloth and fanning. Look for and treat other causes (for example, pneumonia, malaria).

33

TREATMENT PLAN A
TO TREAT DIARRHOEA

EXPLAIN THE THREE RULES FOR TREATING DIARRHOEA AT HOME:

1. GIVE YOUR CHILD MORE FLUIDS THAN USUAL TO PREVENT DEHYDRATION.
   SUITABLE FLUIDS INCLUDE:
   - The recommended home fluid or food-based fluids, such as gruel, soup, or rice water.
   - Breast milk or milk feeds prepared with twice the usual amount of water.

2. GIVE YOUR CHILD FOOD:
   - Give freshly prepared foods. Recommended foods are mixes of cereal and beans, or cereal and meat or fish. Add a few drops of oil to the food, if possible.
   - Give fresh fruit juices or bananas to provide potassium.
   - Offer food every 3 or 4 hours (6 times a day) or more often for very young children.
   - Encourage the child to eat as much as he or she wants.
   - Cook and mash or grind food well so it will be easier to digest.
   - After the diarrhoea stops, give one extra meal each day for a week, or until the child has regained normal weight.

3. TAKE YOUR CHILD TO THE HEALTH WORKER IF THE CHILD HAS ANY OF THE FOLLOWING:
   - passes many stools ⎫
   - is very thirsty   ⎬ These 3 signs suggest your child is dehydrated.
   - has sunken eyes   ⎭
   - has a fever
   - does not eat or drink normally
   - seems not to be getting better.

TEACH THE MOTHER HOW TO USE ORS SOLUTION AT HOME, IF:
   - The mother cannot come back if the diarrhoea gets worse.
   - It is national policy to give ORS to all children who see a health worker for diarrhoea treatment, or
   - Her child has been on Plan B, to prevent dehydration from coming back.

SHOW HER HOW TO MIX AND GIVE ORS.

SHOW HER HOW MUCH TO GIVE:
   - 50-100 ml (¼ to ½ large cup) of ORS solution after each stool for a child under 2 years old.
   - 100-200 ml (½ to 1 large cup) for older children.
   - Adults should drink as much as they want.

TELL HER IF THE CHILD VOMITS, wait 10 minutes. Then continue giving the solution but more slowly — a spoonful every 2-3 minutes.

GIVE HER ENOUGH PACKETS FOR 2 DAYS.

Note: While a child is getting ORS, he or she should be given breast milk or dilute milk feeds and should be offered food. Food-based fluids or a salt and sugar solution should *NOT* be given in addition to ORS.

EXPLAIN HOW SHE CAN PREVENT DIARRHOEA BY:

Giving only breast milk for the first 4-6 months and continuing to breast-feed for at least the first year.

Introducing clean, nutritious weaning foods at 4-6 months.

Giving her child freshly prepared and well-cooked food and clean drinking-water.

Having all family members wash their hands with soap after defecating, and before eating or preparing food.

Having all family members use a latrine.

Quickly disposing of the stool of a young child by putting it into a latrine or by burying it.

TREATMENT PLAN B
TO TREAT DEHYDRATION

1. AMOUNT OF ORS SOLUTION TO GIVE IN FIRST 4 TO 6 HOURS

Patient's age		2 4 6 8 10 12 18 2 3 4 6 8 15					adult
		├──months ──→ ←──years ──→					
Patient's weight in kilograms		3 5 7 9 11 13 15 20 30 40 50					
Give this much solution for 4-6 hours	in ml	200-400	400-600	600-800	800-1000	1000-2000	2000-4000
	in local unit of measure						

- Use the patient's age only when you do not know the weight.

NOTE: ENCOURAGE THE MOTHER TO CONTINUE BREAST-FEEDING.

If the patient wants more ORS, give more.
If the eyelids become puffy, stop ORS and give other fluids. If diarrhoea continues, use ORS again when the puffiness is gone.
If the child vomits, wait 10 minutes and then continue giving ORS, but more slowly.

2. IF THE MOTHER CAN REMAIN AT THE HEALTH CENTRE

- Show her how much solution to give her child.
- Show her how to give it — a spoonful every 1 to 2 minutes.
- Check from time to time to see if she has problems.

3. AFTER 4 TO 6 HOURS, REASSESS THE CHILD USING THE ASSESSMENT CHART. THEN CHOOSE THE SUITABLE TREATMENT PLAN.

Note: If a child will continue on Plan B, tell the mother to offer small amounts of food.

If the child is under 12 months, tell the mother to:
- continue breast-feeding or
- if she does not breast-feed, give 100-200 ml of clean water before continuing ORS.

4. IF THE MOTHER MUST LEAVE ANY TIME BEFORE COMPLETING TREATMENT PLAN B

- Give her enough ORS packets for 2 days and show her how to prepare the fluid.
- Show her how much ORS to give to finish the 4-6 hour treatment at home.
- Tell her to give the child as much ORS and other fluids as he or she wants after the 4-6 hour treatment is finished.
- Tell her to offer the child small amounts of food every 3-4 hours.
- Tell her to bring the child back to the health worker if the child has any of the following:
  - passes many stools ⎱
  - is very thirsty   ⎰ These 3 signs suggest the child is dehydrated.
  - has sunken eyes
  - has a fever
  - does not eat or drink normally
  - seems not to be getting better.

TREATMENT PLAN C
TO TREAT SEVERE
DEHYDRATION QUICKLY

Follow the arrows. If the answer to the questions is 'yes', go across. If it is 'no', go down.

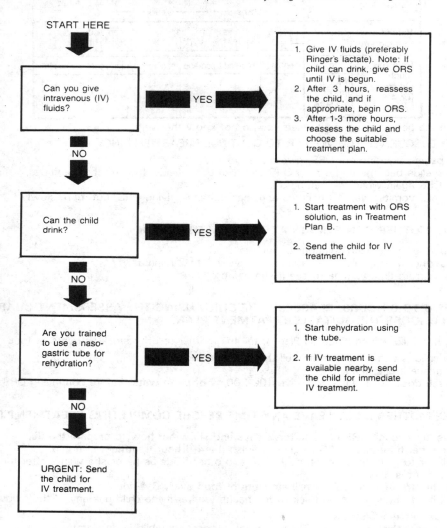

START HERE

Can you give intravenous (IV) fluids?

YES

1. Give IV fluids (preferably Ringer's lactate). Note: If child can drink, give ORS until IV is begun.
2. After 3 hours, reassess the child, and if appropriate, begin ORS.
3. After 1-3 more hours, reassess the child and choose the suitable treatment plan.

NO

Can the child drink?

YES

1. Start treatment with ORS solution, as in Treatment Plan B.
2. Send the child for IV treatment.

NO

Are you trained to use a naso-gastric tube for rehydration?

YES

1. Start rehydration using the tube.
2. If IV treatment is available nearby, send the child for immediate IV treatment.

NO

URGENT: Send the child for IV treatment.

NOTE: If the child is above 2 years of age and cholera is known to be currently occurring in your area, suspect cholera and give an appropriate oral antibiotic once the child is alert.

Annex 2. How to treat diarrhoea at home (Mother's card)

HOW TO TREAT DIARRHOEA AT HOME
1.

AS SOON AS DIARRHOEA STARTS, GIVE YOUR CHILD MORE FLUIDS THAN USUAL TO PREVENT DEHYDRATION. SUITABLE FLUIDS INCLUDE:

- the recommended home fluid or food-based fluids, such as gruel, soup, or rice water.
- breastmilk, or milk feeds prepared with twice the usual amount of water.

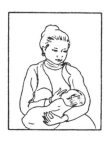 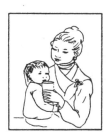

3.
TAKE YOUR CHILD TO THE HEALTH WORKER IF THE CHILD:

- passes many stools ⎫
- is very thirsty ⎬ signs of dehydration
- has sunken eyes ⎭
- has a fever
- does not eat or drink normally
- seems not to be getting better.

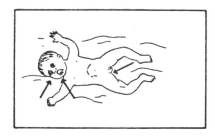

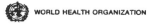 WORLD HEALTH ORGANIZATION

2.
GIVE YOUR CHILD FOOD

- which is freshly prepared, for example, mixes of cereal and beans, or cereal and meat or fish. Add oil to food if possible.
- fresh fruit juices or bananas.
- as much as the child wants, 6 or more times a day.
- which is cooked and mashed or ground well so it will be easier to digest.
- after the diarrhoea stops, one extra meal each day for a week.

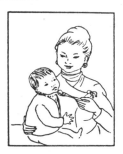

4.
YOU CAN PREVENT DIARRHOEA BY:

- giving only breastmilk for the first 4-6 months and continuing to breastfeed for the first year.
- introducing clean, nutritious weaning foods at 4-6 months.
- giving your child freshly prepared and well-cooked food and clean drinking water.
- having all family members wash their hands with soap after defecating and before eating or preparing food.
- having all family members use a latrine.
- quickly disposing of the stool of a young child in a latrine.

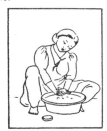

Annex 3. How to tell if a child is undernourished

The upper arm is made up of bone, muscles and fat. When babies are about 1 year old, they have quite a lot of fat under the skin of their arms. By the time they are 5 years old, there is much less fat but more muscle. The distance around the upper arm remains almost the same between the ages of 1 and 5 years.

If a child is undernourished, the amount of muscle and fat in the arm is reduced. The distance around the arm is reduced, and the arm becomes thin. By placing a special arm tape around the upper arm you can find out whether or not a child between the ages of 1 and 5 is undernourished.

This measuring strip is called a tri-coloured arm strip and looks like this:

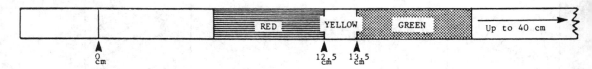

You can make a measuring strip from a piece of string or strip of material that does not stretch, being careful that the markings are accurate.

To use this strip:

Put it around the middle of the upper arm of the child and see which colour is touched by the 0 cm mark on the strip.

- If the green part is touched, the child is well nourished.
- If the yellow part is touched, the child is moderately undernourished.
- If the red part is touched, the child is severely undernourished.

This method is useful because the health worker can identify undernutrition in a child without using a scale or knowing the child's age. However, since it only shows large changes in a child's nutrition, it is not suitable for determining whether the child is improving or becoming worse.

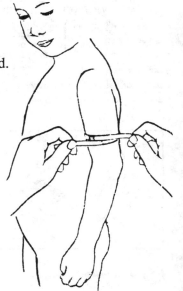

Annex 4. What a health worker should do when packets of oral rehydration salts are not available

The health worker should understand the routine procedure for ordering ORS packets, and the procedure for obtaining emergency supplies quickly. The health worker should also know, according to the national policy, what to do if packets are not available.

1. If packets of ORS are not available, oral rehydration solution can be made with the salts and sugars shown in the following table.

Salts and sugars	Amount required for 1 litre of oral rehydration solution [1]	Note
Sodium chloride (common salt)	3.5 g	You cannot make oral rehydration solution without this.
Glucose or sucrose (common sugar)	20 g 40 g	You cannot make oral rehydration solution without one of these.
Trisodium citrate, dihydrate or sodium bicarbonate	2.9 g 2.5 g	You can make oral rehydration solution without these, but it is much better if you have one, or more, of them.
Potassium chloride	1.5 g	

[1] The sugar and salts (in the amounts shown) should be completely dissolved in one litre of clean drinking-water to make oral rehydration solution. Boiled water, cooled before use, is best.

2. The salts and sugars can be measured by any of the following methods. If you measure the salts and sugars in bulk, it is very important to mix them well before dividing them into smaller amounts.

Method 1
A scale may be available, for example, in a local pharmacy.

Method 2
Small volume measures (such as 5- or 10-ml syringes) can be used to give approximate weights as follows:

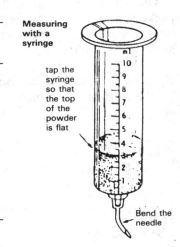

Measuring with a syringe

tap the syringe so that the top of the powder is flat

Bend the needle

Salts and sugars	Approximate weight	Volume
Sodium chloride (common salt)	3.5 g	3 ml
Glucose	20 g	30 ml
Sucrose (common sugar)	40 g	50 ml
Trisodium citrate, dihydrate	2.9 g	3 ml
Sodium bicarbonate	2.5 g	3 ml
Potassium chloride	1.5 g	1.5 ml

Note: The density of an ingredient can vary substantially depending on how the ingredient is made and stored. Therefore, the above volume measurements will not always be an accurate measure of weight.

If health workers do not have a scale and need to use volume measures, it is important to verify exactly what volume corresponds to the necessary weight of each ingredient.

If a precision scale is available, for instance at district level, this should be used to determine the volumes corresponding to the correct weights of each ingredient. The correct volumes should be recorded and this information given to health workers who measure ingredients for ORS.

Whenever ingredients are obtained from a new supplier or manufacturer, the volumes should be checked again.

Method 3
Measuring spoons

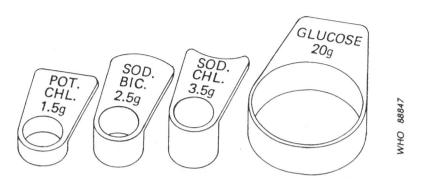

A set of 4 measuring spoons may be ordered from TALC
(Foundation for Teaching Aids at Low Cost), PO Box 49,
St. Albans, Herts AL1 4AX, England.

3. Rehydration solutions that contain sugar and three salts (as described in Point 1 of this Annex) are best. Packets of ORS are most convenient for making oral rehydration solution because the sugar and salts are already measured.

   Other solutions, for example, those made with common salt and sugar only, should be used **only** if ORS packets or all of the ingredients recommended on page 39 are not available.

Annex 5. Oral rehydration using a nasogastric tube

If a health worker is trained to use a nasogastric tube, he or she can give ORS solution to a child who is not in shock but who cannot drink. When a child is in shock, a nasogastric tube should be used only in an emergency (that is, when it is difficult to give intravenous treatment). ORS solution can be put into the nasogastric tube using a syringe or a clean, used, intravenous infusion bottle.

The recommended rate is 20 ml per kg of body weight per hour.

If the patient's abdomen becomes swollen during this treatment, stop giving ORS solution.

Annex 6. Intravenous therapy for severe dehydration

1. The technique of administration

The technique of administration of intravenous fluids can only be taught by practical demonstration by someone with experience. Intravenous therapy should be given only by people who have been trained in the technique. Several general points are made here.

The needles, tubing, bottles, and fluid used for intravenous therapy must be sterile.

Intravenous therapy can be given using any convenient vein. The most accessible veins are generally those in front of the elbow, on the back of the hand, at the ankle, or, in infants, on the side of the scalp.

Use of neck veins or incision to locate a vein is usually not necessary and should be avoided if possible.

In cases requiring rapid resuscitation the femoral vein may be used. In this case, the needle must be held firmly in place and removed as soon as possible. In some cases of severe dehydration, particularly in adults, infusion into two veins may be necessary; one infusion line can be removed once rehydration is well in progress.

It is useful to mark intravenous fluid bottles at various levels with the times at which the fluid should have fallen to those levels. This allows for easier monitoring of the rate of administration.

2. Solutions for intravenous infusion

A number of solutions are available for intravenous infusion; however, some do not contain appropriate or adequate amounts of the electrolytes required to correct the deficits occurring when dehydration is associated with acute diarrhoea. The following is a brief discussion of the relative suitability of each of the available solutions.

Preferred solution

Ringer's lactate solution. This is also called Hartmann's solution for injection. It is the best commercially available solution. It supplies adequate concentrations of sodium and potassium, and the lactate yields bicarbonate for correction of acidosis (a condition resulting from a relative excess of acid in the blood, in the case of diarrhoea, primarily due to loss of alkali in the stool). It can be used in all age groups to treat dehydration due to acute diarrhoea of any cause.

Less suitable solutions

ORS solution given by nasogastric tube should be considered as an alternative to the use of the following intravenous solutions. If any of these solutions are used, they should be replaced by ORS solution given by mouth as soon as the patient can drink.

Half-strength Darrow's solution. This is also called lactated potassic saline. This solution does not contain enough sodium chloride to correct the sodium deficit and ongoing sodium losses found in adults with severe dehydration and continuing severe diarrhoea.

Normal saline. This is also called isotonic or physiological saline. This solution is often readily available. It will not correct acidosis and will not replace potassium losses. Sodium bicarbonate or sodium lactate and potassium chloride can be given at the same time, but this requires careful calculation of amounts, and monitoring is difficult.

Half-normal saline in 5% dextrose. Like normal saline, this solution will not correct acidosis or replace potassium losses. It also will not provide enough sodium chloride for many adults with acute diarrhoea.

Unsuitable solutions

Plain glucose and dextrose solutions. These should not be used as they provide only water and sugar. They do not contain electrolytes and thus they do not correct the electrolyte loss or the acidosis.

3. Providing intravenous therapy for severe dehydration

The purpose is to give the patient a large quantity of fluid quickly to replace the very large fluid loss which has resulted in severe dehydration.

Begin intravenous therapy quickly, giving the amounts specified in the table on the following page.

Guidelines for rehydration therapy for severe dehydration [1]

Age group	Type of fluid and route of administration	Amount of fluid (ml per kg of body weight)	Time of administration
Infants (under 12 months) Ringer's lactate, intravenously	30	Within 1 hour	
	Followed by		
	Ringer's lactate, intravenously	40	Within next 2 hours
	Followed by (if appropriate)		
	ORS solution, orally	40	Within next 3 hours
Other children and adults	Ringer's lactate, intravenously	100	Within 3 hours; initially as fast as possible until radial pulse is easily felt

[1] The volumes of fluid and rates of administration are averages based on usual needs. These amounts should be increased if they are not adequate to achieve rehydration, or decreased if rehydration is achieved earlier than expected, or if the appearance of puffiness around the eyes suggests overhydration. Once the health worker has gained some experience in rehydration therapy he or she may not need to follow this exact schedule.

For an infant who is severely dehydrated, the entire 6-hour course of therapy should be followed to restore quickly the fluid loss. During the 6-hour period, the progess of the rehydration therapy should be assessed after one hour and then every 1–2 hours to determine whether the volume or rate of administration needs to be increased.

In particular, attention should be given to:
— the number and volume of stools passed
— the extent of vomiting
— the presence of, and changes in, the signs of dehydration
— whether the rehydration fluid (oral or intravenous) is being successfully given, and in adequate amounts.

If the signs of dehydration and the diarrhoea and vomiting become worse, or remain unchanged, the rate of administration and the amount of fluid given may need to be increased.

While rehydration therapy (to replace the body's abnormal loss of fluid) is in progress, the patient's normal daily fluid requirements must also be considered. As soon as an infant can suck, begin breast-feeding again. After 6 hours, give non-breast-fed infants 100–200 ml of clean water before continuing with oral rehydration therapy. For older children and adults, plain water, in addition to oral rehydration solution, should be available to patients to drink as and when they wish.

After the first 6 hours (3 hours for older children and adults), ASK, LOOK, and FEEL again for the signs of dehydration as described on pages 9–11. At this point complete, or nearly complete, rehydration of the severely dehydrated patient should have been achieved. To prevent dehydration returning, the patient will require continued therapy for as long as the diarrhoea continues.

- If no signs of dehydration remain, use Treatment Plan A — *To treat diarrhoea.*
- If some of the signs of dehydration are still present, but the child is improving, give ORS for another 6 hours in the amount specified in the table in Treatment Plan B.
- If the signs of dehydration are worse, or remain unchanged, rehydration therapy must be continued.

Annex 7. Antibiotics used to treat diarrhoea caused by specific illnesses

Cause of diarrhoea	Antibiotics of choice [1]	Alternative antibiotics [1]
Cholera [2,3]	Tetracycline *Children*: 50 mg per kg of body weight per day, divided into 4 doses, for 2 days. *Adults*: 500 mg, 4 times a day, for 3 days.	Furazolidone *Children*: 5 mg per kg of body weight, per day, divided into 4 doses, for 3 days. *Adults*: 100 mg, 4 times a day, for 3 days. Trimethoprim and sulfa-methoxazole [4] *All ages*: 8 mg of trimethoprim per kg of body weight per day *and* 40 mg of sulfamethoxazole per kg of body weight, per day, each divided into 2 doses, for 3 days.
Shigella dysentery [2]	Trimethoprim and sulfamethoxazole *Children*: 10 mg trimethoprim per kg of body weight, per day *and* 50 mg of sulfamethoxazole per kg of body weight per day, each divided into 2 doses, for 5 days. *Adults*: 160 mg of trimethoprim *and* 800 mg of sulfamethoxazole twice daily, for 5 days. *or* Nalidixic acid *Children*: 55 mg per kg of body weight, per day, divided into 4 doses, for 5 days. *Adults*: 1 g, 3 times a day, for 5 days.	

[1, 2, 3, 4] See notes on page 48.

¹ All doses given are for oral administration. If drugs are not available in liquid form for use in young children, tablets should be divided as accurately as possible to obtain the required doses.

² The selection of antibiotics for treatment should take into account the frequency of resistance to antibiotics in the area.

³ Antibiotic therapy is not essential for successful therapy, but it shortens the duration of illness and the excretion of disease-causing organisms in severe cases.

⁴ Other choices of antibiotic include chloramphenicol, to be given in the same dosages as tetracycline, and erythromycin — 30 mg per kg of body weight per day, divided into 3 doses, for 3 days. Adults — 250 mg, every 6 hours.

Annex 8. Check-list of points of essential skills and knowledge

In order to prevent and treat acute diarrhoea, a health worker should be able to:

- Define diarrhoea in a way that is appropriate to his or her work setting.
- Distinguish between acute and chronic diarrhoea.
- Explain why diarrhoea is dangerous.
- Explain how diarrhoea causes dehydration.
- Describe the most important parts of the treatment of diarrhoea.
- Explain to family members the three rules for home treatment of diarrhoea. These are: to increase fluids; to continue to feed the child; and to take a child who is not getting better to the health worker.
- Ask, look, and feel for signs of dehydration, and check for problems other than dehydration.
- Select the appropriate Treatment Plan using the Assessment Chart given on page 10, and in Annex 1.
- Demonstrate how to prepare ORS solution correctly.
- Give oral rehydration therapy to children with dehydration.
- Give intravenous rehydration therapy to children with severe dehydration or refer them for this treatment.
- Teach mothers how to continue treatment at home.
- Keep appropriate records of the treatment given.
- Describe what families can do to prevent diarrhoea, including: breast-feeding; improved weaning practices; the use of plenty of clean water; hand-washing; the use of latrines; proper disposal of the stools of young children; and immunization against measles.
- List several things that health workers can do to support preventive practices.

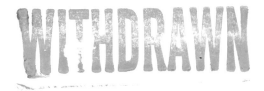

WHO publications may be obtained, direct or through booksellers, from:

ALGERIA : Entreprise nationale du Livre (ENAL), 3 bd Zirout Youcef, ALGIERS

ARGENTINA : Carlos Hirsch, SRL, Florida 165, Galerías Güemes, Escritorio 453/465, BUENOS AIRES

AUSTRALIA : Hunter Publications, 58A Gipps Street, COLLINGWOOD, VIC 3066.

AUSTRIA : Gerold & Co., Graben 31, 1011 VIENNA I

BAHRAIN : United Schools International, Arab Region Office, P.O. Box 726, BAHRAIN

BANGLADESH : The WHO Representative, G.P.O. Box 250, DHAKA 5

BELGIUM : *For books :* Office International de Librairie s.a., avenue Marnix 30, 1050 BRUSSELS. *For periodicals and subscriptions :* Office International des Périodiques, avenue Louise 485, 1050 BRUSSELS.

BHUTAN : *see* India, WHO Regional Office

BOTSWANA : Botsalo Books (Pty) Ltd., P.O. Box 1532, GABORONE

BRAZIL : Centro Latinoamericano de Informação em Ciencias de Saúde (BIREME), Organização Panamericana de Saúde, Sector de Publicações, C.P. 20381 - Rua Botucatu 862, 04023 SÃO PAULO, SP

BURMA : *see* India, WHO Regional Office

CAMEROON : Cameroon Book Centre, P.O. Box 123, South West Province, VICTORIA

CANADA : Canadian Public Health Association, 1335 Carling Avenue, Suite 210, OTTAWA, Ont. K1Z 8N8. (Tel : (613) 725–3769. Telex : 21–053–3841)

CHINA : China National Publications Import & Export Corporation, P.O. Box 88, BEIJING (PEKING)

DEMOCRATIC PEOPLE'S REPUBLIC OF KOREA : *see* India, WHO Regional Office

DENMARK : Munksgaard Export and Subscription Service, Nørre Søgade 35, 1370 COPENHAGEN K (Tel : + 45 1 12 85 70)

FIJI : The WHO Representative, P.O. Box 113, SUVA

FINLAND : Akateeminen Kirjakauppa, Keskuskatu 2, 00101 HELSINKI 10

FRANCE : Arnette, 2 rue Casimir-Delavigne, 75006 PARIS

GERMAN DEMOCRATIC REPUBLIC : Buchhaus Leipzig, Postfach 140, 701 LEIPZIG

GERMANY FEDERAL REPUBLIC OF : Govi-Verlag GmbH, Ginnheimerstrasse 20, Postfach 5360, 6236 ESCHBORN — Buchhandlung Alexander Horn, Kirchgasse 22, Postfach 3340, 6200 WIESBADEN

GREECE : G.C. Eleftheroudakis S.A., Librairie internationale, rue Nikis 4, 105-63 ATHENS

HONG KONG : Hong Kong Government Information Services, Publication (Sales) Office, Information Services Department, No. 1, Battery Path, Central, HONG KONG.

HUNGARY : Kultura, P.O.B. 149, BUDAPEST 62

ICELAND : Snaebjorn Jonsson & Co., Hafnarstraeti 9, P.O. Box 1131, IS-101 REYKJAVIK

INDIA : WHO Regional Office for South-East Asia, World Health House, Indraprastha Estate, Mahatma Gandhi Road, NEW DELHI 110002

IRAN (ISLAMIC REPUBLIC OF) : Iran University Press, 85 Park Avenue, P.O. Box 54/551, TEHERAN

IRELAND : TDC Publishers, 12 North Frederick Street, DUBLIN 1 (Tel : 744835–749677)

ISRAEL : Heiliger & Co., 3 Nathan Strauss Street, JERUSALEM 94227

ITALY : Edizioni Minerva Medica, Corso Bramante 83–85, 10126 TURIN ; Via Lamarmora 3, 20100 MILAN ; Via Spallanzani 9, 00161 ROME

JAPAN : Maruzen Co. Ltd., P.O. Box 5050, TOKYO International, 100–31

JORDAN : Jordan Book Centre Co. Ltd., University Street, P.O. Box 301 (Al-Jubeiha), AMMAN

KENYA : Text Book Centre Ltd, P.O. Box 47540, NAIROBI

KUWAIT : The Kuwait Bookshops Co. Ltd., Thunayan Al-Ghanem Bldg, P.O. Box 2942, KUWAIT

LAO PEOPLE'S DEMOCRATIC REPUBLIC : The WHO Representative, P.O. Box 343, VIENTIANE

LUXEMBOURG : Librairie du Centre, 49 bd Royal, LUXEMBOURG

A/1/88